Intermittent] For Beginners

A Simple 21-Day Beginners Guide to Fast Weight Loss, Fat Burn and Long Term Health

© Copyright 2018 - All rights reserved.

The contents of this book may not be reproduced, duplicated or transmitted without direct written permission from the author.

Under no circumstances will any legal responsibility or blame be held against the publisher for any reparation, damages, or monetary loss due to the information herein, either directly or indirectly.

Legal Notice:

You cannot amend, distribute, sell, use, quote or paraphrase any part or the content within this book without the consent of the author.

Disclaimer Notice:

Please note the information contained within this document is for educational and entertainment purposes only. No warranties of any kind are expressed or implied. Readers acknowledge that the author is not engaging in the rendering of legal, financial, medical or professional advice. Please consult a licensed professional before attempting any techniques outlined in this book.

By reading this document, the reader agrees that under no circumstances are is the author responsible for any losses, direct or indirect, which are incurred as a result of the use of information contained within this document, including, but not limited to, —errors, omissions, or inaccuracies.

Table of Contents

Introduction 1
Chapter One: Basics of Intermittent Fasting 2
    Fasting 3
Chapter Two: Methods of Intermittent Fasting 6
    Warrior diet 6
    16/8 method 7
    5:2 Diet 7
    Eat-stop-Eat 8
    Skipping meals spontaneously 9
    Alternate day fasting 10
Chapter Three: Benefits 11
    Benefits your skin 11
    Improved breathing 11
    Oxidative stress in the body 12
    Reduces Inflammation 12
    Good for your Brain's Health 13
    Cellular Repair 13
Chapter Four: Process 14
    Check with your doctor 15
    Trust the process 15
    Start cutting down on the snacks 16
    Don't dive right in 16
    Sip on a lot of hot drinks 17

Stay focused 17
Tone down your workouts 18

Chapter Five: How to Make Intermittent Fasting work in 21-days..20

Dos and Don'ts during fasting 20
Blend fasting with your daily lifestyle 20
Don't overeat your last meal 21
Prepare yourself well 21
Don't take up any rigorous exercise routines 22
Remember to take your vitamins 22
Hydrate well 23
Hunt for fun distractions 23
Take help from your friends 24
Don't stress 24
Avoid the victory binge 25

Conclusion 26

Introduction

Losing weight seems like a ginormous task and when there are multiple diets and methods that are publicized as 'the best way of losing weight,' it's hard to figure out what strategy is right. Of course, the one advice that is common among all these weight loss strategies is to eat less. Eating less can simply be seen as a way to reduce your food portion which, in turn, will push your body to use the fats stored in your body. This can work no doubt, but it's a long process and it might not turn out to be as effective as you thought.

This is where fasting comes in; fasting is something that has been followed in many cultures around the world and they swear by its effectiveness. The basic goal of fasting is to make your body use stored fat, but it tries to make the process faster.

Intermittent Fasting has only one goal, which is to make sure that you lose weight as quickly as possible while getting the right nutrition for your body. It's a system where there are set periods of times within which you can eat a certain amount of calories, while you starve yourself for the rest of the time. There are many variations of this process and hence, many different methods have popped up, each with a different time schedule. The most common one is the 16:8 method where you eat within a set period of 8 hours and fast for the rest of the time.

Intermittent Fasting is not just a new trend but has a lot of scientific basis for why it's effective. In this book, we're going to look at what exactly intermittent fasting is, how it works, its benefits and how you can follow it.

Let us get started and read all about it!

Chapter One
Basics of Intermittent Fasting

What time do you generally have your dinner? It must be around 8 pm in all probability. What time do you have your breakfast? Do you grab a cup of coffee with a couple of slices of toast at around 7 or 8 am just before leaving for work? If your answer is affirmative, you have just found the reason why you are unable to keep your weight under control. As per scientific evidence, intermittent fasting is linked with weight loss as well as hormonal control. More and more people are trying to prolong the time when they do not eat. Forget calorie counting, eliminating carbs from your diet or giving up on your favourite foods. All you may need for weight loss is to eat for fewer hours every day.

Intermittent fasting proposes eating enough for eight hours a day and going without food for the next 16 hours. You can eat all the food you wish to eat within those eight hours. For instance, you can start your day by eating breakfast at 10.00 AM and consume the final meal of your day by around 6 PM. Now how many calories you consume within this eight-hour period is not important. What's important is that you allow your body to digest the food within the next 16 hours properly. You don't have to change your habits drastically; rather you can go slow and then gradually increase the number of hours within which you don't eat anything.

There were various studies conducted on rats using intermittent fasting where they were fed high-fat foods but only for a shorter period. These studies showed that they weighed less, had no cholesterol issues or inflammation in their bodies. On the other hand, some rats were allowed to eat throughout the day and developed high cholesterol and a fatty liver. Researchers came to the conclusion that when the body is frequently fed, the insulin levels go up, and people end up putting on weight and stressing their livers. However, when we go without food for longer periods, our body's natural repairing mechanism works more efficiently, which in turn keeps it functioning well. It also prevents our liver from releasing excessive glucose into the bloodstream, thereby reducing inflammation.

In real life, this plan may seem a little impossible considering our hectic schedules, which result in the consumption of snacks throughout the day or night. Our environment encourages regular consumption of food, regardless of whether you are hungry or not. If 16 hours seem too difficult to follow, for starters, you can try going 12 hours without food. You can indeed gorge on snacks as well, but just make sure that you consume them in the 12-hour period and go completely without food for the next 12. One of the biggest issues with diets is that they leave you feeling hungry all the time. To avoid this, ensure that your final meal is substantial enough to keep you satiated for the next 12 hours.

Fasting

The concept of fasting isn't a new one, and human beings have been doing this forever. It could have been done out of necessity or due to the lack of food. There are religious reasons for fasting too. Various religions like Islam, Hinduism, Buddhism, and Christianity, talk about fasting. Animals and human beings alike tend to fast when they fall sick. There isn't anything that is unnatural or unusual about fasting, and our bodies have been designed in such a way that they can go for long periods of time without any food. Different processes in our bodies also change when we start fasting. The level of blood sugar, as well as insulin, tends to drop down while fasting and there is an increase in the production of the growth hormone in the body. People follow intermittent fasting since it allows them to shed weight and it is quite an easy way to achieve that goal. Others follow this diet for the metabolic benefits that it has to offer. There's some research that suggests that this diet can help in providing some protection against diseases that affect the heart and the brain.

Fasting has many benefits to offer, that go well beyond weight loss. Fasting can help in improving your overall health and improve the longevity of your life as well. In a recent study that was conducted to study the link between cell metabolism and fasting, it was found that fasting periodically can help in decreasing the risk of heart disease, diabetes, ageing and so on. Fasting is effective, as, during this period, a lot of cells that are present in the body die and the stem cells start working. This starts the regeneration process and produces new cells. Other studies also show that it helps in reducing the amount of bad cholesterol or LDL present in the blood.

Also, given these benefits, it is safe to conclude that fasting can help you be healthy and actually live longer. So, going without food sometimes will make you healthier and stronger. This diet doesn't place any caloric constraint on those who follow it. The plans for this diet can be personalized quite easily. It focuses more on the time at which you can eat and not what you eat. The food doesn't matter. What matters is that you adhere to the fasting window. This diet might not work for everyone. Don't get disheartened; you can try a different variation of the same diet. Also, before you get started with this diet, you should consult your physician or your doctor.

Intermittent fasting seems like a handy tip that will make your life much simpler, and improve your health simultaneously. The fewer meals you have to plan, the easier your life will be.

Intermittent fasting might mean different things to different people. The most common form of the diet is the 5:2 model. In this method, the individual will have to fast for two non consecutive days in the week. The rest of the days, there is no restriction on the number of calories that you can consume. There are others who might fast daily and have a fasting window that fits in with their schedule. This is like the 16/8 pattern. This means that you will have to skip your breakfast, have your first meal at noon and the last one before 8 pm.

Chapter Two
Methods of Intermittent Fasting

Intermittent fasting has become quite trendy in the recent past. It offers a wide range of benefits. Given its popularity, there are different variations of intermittent fasting that have been cropping up. All these methods can be effective; however, there will be one out of the lot that will fit the needs of an individual better than another. Let us take a look at the most popular methods of intermittent fasting.

Warrior diet

Ori Hofmekler is responsible for popularizing this diet, and he is a well-renowned fitness expert. This form of fasting involves the consumption of small quantities of raw fruit and veggies during the day and then consuming a single hearty meal at night. Essentially, you will need to fast throughout the day, and then you get to feast at night. The feeding window extends to only 4 hours. This variation of the intermittent fasting diet was one of the first ones to be popular. While following this method of fasting, the food choices that you make should be quite similar to what you would have made had you been following the Paleo diet. You will need to consume foods that are unprocessed. You can eat anything that our cavemen ancestors would have consumed.

16/8 method

This method prescribes that an individual should fast for a period of 16 hours every day. The eating window is restricted to about 8-10 hours. Within this window, you can manage to squeeze in two or three meals. This is also known as Lean gains, and it was made popular by Martin Berkhan, a fitness expert. It could be something as simple as skipping breakfast or not munching on anything after dinner. For instance, you can make sure that the last meal that you have is at 8 in the evening. Make sure that you don't eat anything until noon the following day. This provides you with a fasting window of about 16 hours. It has been observed that it would be better for women to fast for a shorter duration of time and don't let their fasting period go beyond 14-15 hours. For those who feel hungry in the morning and are used to having breakfast every day, this can be hard initially. However, if you were already used to skipping breakfast, then it would be easy. You can have water, coffee, and other beverages that don't have any calories in them while you are fasting. It is important that you stay away from all forms of junk food and eat healthy during the fast. This diet won't work out if you binge on foods that have a high caloric value. It will be easier to stick to intermittent fasting if you consume low-calorie meals.

5:2 Diet

While following this diet, the individual gets to eat normally for five days of the week and restricts the calorie intake to 500-600 calories on the other two days of the week. This diet is referred to as the Fast diet and was made popular by

Michael Mosley, a British doctor, and journalist. On the two fasting days, it is recommended that women should have 500 calories and men can consume 600 calories. For instance, you get to eat normally on all days except the two days when you want to fast. On such days, you can eat two meals consisting of 250-300 calories each depending on your gender. This diet is suitable for all those who feel that they cannot fast for the whole day and who would like to eat a little something.

Eat-stop-Eat

This form of intermittent fasting requires the individual to fast for 24 hours, once or twice every week. Brad Pilon, a fitness expert, popularized this diet a few years ago. You will need to fast for 24 hours in this diet. From dinner on one day until dinner the consecutive day, that would constitute 24 hours. For instance, you had your dinner at 7 pm on Monday and you don't get to eat until 7 pm on Tuesday. This would be the 24 hours fasting window. You can also do this from breakfast on a given day until breakfast on the following day. You will just need to fast for 24 hours; you can select the timings according to your convenience. You cannot consume any solid food during this diet. However, water, coffee, and other beverages that don't have any calories in them can be safely consumed. If you are following this method because you want to lose weight, then in such a case you will need to eat normally during your feeding window. You should eat the sort of food you are used to eating, had you not been fasting. The only problem with this method is that there happens to be a 24-hour fasting window and it might be difficult for a few people to follow. You don't have to necessarily start out with this. You can gradually progress from the 16-hour fasting model. The first stretch of the diet won't be hard; it is only towards the end that this diet gets a little difficult to follow. This is where discipline and motivation will come in handy.

Skipping meals spontaneously

There is no structured plan for this form of intermittent fasting. You can reap all the benefits offered by an intermittent fast without having to plan any elaborate meals. This is quite an easy variation to follow. You will simply have to skip meals spontaneously from time to time. Skip meals whenever you aren't hungry or you are preoccupied with some work. It definitely is a myth that people will need to eat every couple of hours. Your body won't start losing muscle or even shift into starvation mode if you go without food for a couple of hours. Our bodies have been designed in such a manner that we can go without food for prolonged periods of time. Missing one or two meals from time to time will not do your body any harm. In fact, it will give your body a break and provide you with an opportunity to cleanse itself. So, if you aren't hungry, you can skip one meal. Then, depending on your hunger quotient, you can have a hearty lunch or dinner accordingly. However, you will need to make sure that the other meals that you are consuming are healthy.

Alternate day fasting

Like the name suggests, this diet is all about fasting on every alternate day. There are different variations of this diet. Some variations allow you to eat about 500 calories on every alternate day, and the others require you to observe a strict fast on every alternate day. Most of the lab studies that have been conducted to find the benefits of intermittent fasting have made use of some variation of this diet. A strict fast might sound rather severe and extreme. Depending upon your comfort level, you can adapt this diet to suit your needs. It is advisable that beginners don't immediately jump to this method. With this method of fasting, be prepared to go to bed hungry a few times every week. This diet doesn't show any form of sustainability in the long run.

Chapter Three
Benefits

Apart from helping you lose weight, intermittent fasting has a truckload health benefits that are mentioned below:

Benefits your skin

A lot of people who have taken to intermittent fasting have reported positive effects on their skin. Throughout my teens, I suffered from several skin issues such as acne, oily skin, and breakouts. Once I started eating my meals for limited hours in a day, my skin changed drastically. But once I got back to eating an early breakfast or having a late night meal, I would experience breakouts again. Eventually, I concluded that the result I was getting earlier was only because of the fasting. When you allow your body an extended break from the digestion routine, it kick-starts your body's detox mechanism too. It also helps your body in digesting the food better and allows it to de-stress. As a result of all this, your skin starts glowing, and you naturally get rid of all skin-related problems.

Improved breathing

You may not think that poor breathing may affect you until you face a respiratory issue. For some years, I struggled with shortness of breath. I consulted my doctor to check if I had asthma, but the reports were negative. Initially, I thought it was my weight that's affecting my breathing. So I started following some fad diets and ended up feeling all the sicker. Not being able to breathe well can make your life miserable and I was feeling stuck. Slowly, I started cutting down on all the dairy and gluten from my diet and started taking vitamin b12 shots. Along with that, I started intermittent fasting, and my breathing got better and better. Today, I no longer suffer from shortness of breath except if I am suffering from severe colds.

Oxidative stress in the body

Do you know that as we breathe, our bodies produce free radicals? A decent and healthy level is fine, as they stimulate repair, but when our body produces more than it should, it may cause damage to our cells – this is called oxidative stress. It is one of the factors for ageing, wrinkles, graying hair and also arthritis.

Several studies have concluded that intermittent fasting may improve the resistance of our body to oxidative stress. Oxidative stress is a process that eventually leads to the destruction of essential molecules in the body through reactions with other unstable molecules such as free radicals. Also, there are more facts and evidence showing that intermittent fasting can help fight inflammation, which is a common cause of many chronic diseases.

Reduces Inflammation

One of the primary reasons for inflammation is excessive free radicals in your body resulting in cellular damage. When mitochondria, the batteries in our cells that give us energy are damaged, they start releasing excessive free radicals. These, in turn, result in inflammation and DNA damage. All these problems automatically vanish when you allow your body to be in the fasted state for extended hours. Fasting controls the release of free radicals present in your body, and thus protects you from inflammation. Those who eat throughout the day are also consuming excessive amounts of salt, which is responsible for bloating in your body. Fasting for prolonged hours along with ample of water consumption can ensure that you may never have to face inflammation issues again.

Good for your Brain's Health

Intermittent fasting improves processes known to be very important for our brain health. It causes reduced inflammation, reduced oxidative stress and reduction in blood sugar levels and insulin resistance. It also eventually increases the levels of a brain-driven neurotrophic factor, a brain hormone whose deficiency is linked to depression & other similar problems of the brain.

Cellular Repair

Fasting also leads to autophagy, which is a cellular process for removal of waste. This entails cells breaking down and also metabolizing dysfunctional, broken proteins, which build up in cells with the passage of time. During this process, your body builds protection against several diseases like Alzheimer's disease & also cancer.

Chapter Four
Process

For some people, the very idea of going without food more than a few hours is terrifying. Now there could be different reasons why they wouldn't readily want to commit to such a diet. It could be because they are used to regularly consuming food, due to some medical conditions or because of their hectic work schedules. However, unless you are suffering from a serious medical condition and you explicitly been told by your physician to eat frequently, there's no reason why you can't follow this diet. Some people are worried about the irritability, hunger pangs or mood swings they might experience if they take up this fasting method. But the truth is far from this. As a matter of fact, people who start following this diet plan often feel fuller, experience fewer mood swings than usual and end up feeling incredibly lighter, which in turn leaves them feeling extremely positive towards life in general.

If you look around, you will find many lean individuals, who are conscious of the calorie consumption, that skip their meals to maintain their weight. As human beings, it's a little challenging to exercise complete restraint over food, but we can certainly control how frequently we consume food. If you are a beginner and are wondering how to go ahead with this type of fasting, we have some valuable tips for you below.

Check with your doctor

Although anyone and everyone regardless of their age can follow intermittent fasting, it's important to check with your doctor if you have any underlying medical conditions. If you are already suffering from a serious ailment or you are pregnant, it's even more vital that you consult your physician before you start with this type of fasting. If you have been under a lot of mental and physical stress lately, then it's advisable that you work on reducing your stress levels first and then start with intermittent fasting. One of the best ways to lead a stress-free lifestyle is to stay away from your phone or social media for a few days and spend some quality time with your loved ones. Sometimes a little "me" time or feeling loved by your family is all it takes to reduce the stress in your life. Once you feel that your body and mind can handle intermittent fasting, you can start off.

Trust the process

Blame it on our conditioning that we have to eat after every few hours that some of us start questioning the process. When we start intermittent fasting, the questions that often start popping up in our head are "Am I starving my body when it should be fed all the time?" Or "Is skipping breakfast a good idea? I mean, after all, it's supposed to be the most important meal of the day." If you catch yourself thinking on these lines, immediately remind yourself that these statements are not necessarily accurate and you need to stick to your plan no matter what. Another thing to remember is not to track your progress every day and make it an excuse for you to fall back into your old ways. Any diet plan or fasting requires a certain amount of time for it to start working. If you are obsessed about tracking your progress every single day, it's only going to discourage you when you don't see results that quickly.

Start cutting down on the snacks

Have you ever noticed the number of snacks we consume even when we aren't hungry? Snacking is more of a habit than a necessity. And what do we snack on? Fried or processed foods, which only put our bodies at a greater risk of obesity. So all the unhealthy trash needs to go right away. When you start having three large meals, which will keep you satiated for longer periods, you will not have to keep snacking. These meals will also keep you energized throughout the day, and you will experience almost no hunger pangs. When your body starts adjusting itself to long periods of fasting, your natural insulin levels, as well as the hormone cycle, begin to function properly. Once you find it easier to control your urge for snacking you will notice how light your body starts feeling.

Don't dive right in

Just start by cutting all kinds of snacks from your daily routine. If you do want something, you can drink a few cups of plain black coffee, which has no caloric value. If you are used to having breakfast, abruptly eliminating it may not seem possible. Instead, you can delay having your breakfast a bit every day. You can start your day at 10 am by having your breakfast and adjust the rest of the meals within the next 8-hour eating period. Breakfast does not necessarily have to be consumed early in the morning; you can eat it slightly later in the day and still maintain your fasted state for longer. Similarly, if you have your final meal at 8 or 9 pm, your best bet would be to consume it about an hour early and then start. If you get all excited and start making a sudden switch, chances are that you may not be able to stick with the fasting for long.

Sip on a lot of hot drinks

The best part about this type of fasting is that you are allowed to sip on any of your favourite beverages minus the added sugar. If you chose to add milk to any of these beverages, make sure that you are adding low-calorie skimmed milk. You can feel free to sip on different types of green teas, herbal tea, plain black coffee, etc. If you find it difficult to sip on unsweetened drinks, you can always use a few drops of Stevia to add some sweetness. However, consuming sugar is a complete no-no, as it's known to add a lot of empty calories to your diet and gets stored in your body in the form of fat. When consumed in excess, it is likely to enter your bloodstream, putting you at a high risk of developing diabetes. Sipping on low-calorie drinks during your fasted state can distract you from wanting to snack and keep you refreshed.

Stay focused

No matter what, don't cave in! Remember what you are fasting for when feel like giving up. You may have taken up to intermittent fasting for weight loss, to detox your body or simply to feel lighter. You need to remind yourself what it is that you are aiming for through this type of fasting. An excellent way to stay focused would be to write down the reasons why you are fasting and read them before you start your day. By doing this, you will program yourself to concentrate on what you are aiming for rather than caving in during the process. On the occasions that you fail to keep up with the fast, don't beat yourself up about it. It's okay not to have the complete willpower to stick to this fasting plan. However, ensure that you get back on track without wasting too much time dwelling on it. Just start over the very next day and know that you can achieve whatever goals you have set for yourself. If you are lacking the necessary motivation, head over to some YouTube channels and Instagram accounts of people who are following the same method of fasting. You will be surprised how easy it is to stay motivated when you are following some inspiring people on social media. That way you will also learn a few more tips as to how you can make this diet more efficient.

Tone down your workouts

Often times, potency requires minimalism. Much like the strength of coffee or any alcoholic drink dissipates as you dilute it with water, the efficacy of your workouts during intermittent fasting may follow suit if you train too much. But what do we mean by over-training in this context?

The obvious examples are exercising at a very high intensity and for more extended periods of time. When you exert too much effort (intensity) than what your body can currently handle, under a fasting state, you run the risk of burning out, getting sick or being injured. Even at the right intensity, regularly working out significantly longer than your body can safely handle runs the same risk as excess intensity. Can you imagine if you do both at the same time?

What is the right intensity? Generally speaking, you'd feel very uncomfortable – light headed, very tired and weak or prolonged muscle soreness – during or after working out if you over-train. A relatively objective way of determining if you're exercising at moderate intensity, which is ideal, is through the talk test. If you can still carry a normal conversation while working out, albeit with some difficulty, that's moderate. If you're able to carry on a conversation in the same manner as you would over coffee with a friend or if you can barely say a word while catching your breath, then you are under (low intensity) or over (high intensity) training, respectively.

A good way to focus your training is to prioritize compound exercises, i.e., those that involve the most major muscle groups to execute the movements. Examples of these would be burpees, which recruit most of your major muscle groups.

Another way of prioritizing your exercise is to go for those that utilize the large muscle groups, particularly legs. Why? The bigger the muscles, the more calories are required to contract them. That's why doing 1,000 crunches aren't enough to get you ripped, but running daily for at least 30 minutes, which involves the biggest muscle group that's the legs, can help you do so.

Chapter Five
How to Make Intermittent Fasting work in 21-days

Dos and Don'ts during fasting

Fasting isn't an entirely new concept as some people might think; it has regularly been practised by various religions across centuries. However, it has just recently experienced a renaissance especially among those who are very health conscious and look at it as some kind of detox mechanism. While it's true that fasting can have a detoxification effect on your body, it also helps you look and feel better too. Unlike during the olden days, where people would go for days without eating, the modern day intermittent fasting options are of a shorter span. They can range from 8 to 36 hours. You can also choose to fast for a longer duration if your body permits. Regardless of the method you choose, you need to know some basic tips so you can sail through the process smoothly. Have you ever considered fasting before? If not, now is the right time to take up this challenge. But before you start your diet plan, take a look at some dos and don'ts when it comes to intermittent fasting.

Blend fasting with your daily lifestyle

Plan your meals before you decide to take up fasting. Don't just randomly start consuming one meal a day during stressful times. This can cause excessive exertion and result in loss of energy. Ensure that your schedule is easy so that the sudden change does not affect you. If you are new to fasting, I highly recommend starting with the 5:2 diet. This type of plan generally works for beginners. Some people like to fast on weekdays and some on the weekends. Whatever you chose, remember to keep your routine stress free.

Don't overeat your last meal

We get it, the idea of fasting may make you feel like stuffing yourself with a large "final meal," but nutritionists say that it could be detrimental to your progress. Most dieticians suggest eating a meal with a lot of healthy fat, lean proteins and plenty of vegetables. You can also include some legumes or even a sweet potato. Including some fruit into your meals can provide your body with some natural sugar and thereby helps in curbing your sugar cravings. Low-glycemic fruit such as berries can be consumed in moderation. Such type of meal provides your body with ample of nutrition so you can carry out your fasting period as smoothly as possible.

Prepare yourself well

It is essential that you are well rested and mentally prepared to take on a sudden change of diet. An emotionally healthy person can easily sail through the initial food cravings that may arise. Along with that, you will also have to ensure that you keep all temptations at bay. Start by clearing your kitchen of any type of processed foods or sugary drinks. Any unhealthy food items need to be eliminated right away. When it comes to fasting, "out of sight is out of mind" is a mantra that can work in your favor. This will undoubtedly help you in focusing on your fasting goals.

Don't take up any rigorous exercise routines

Thinking of running a 5-mile marathon? That is a complete NO during fasting, especially if you are a beginner. Instead, you can perform some light exercise like walking or yoga. Any kind of high-intensity cardiovascular workout during your fasted state will only end up making your muscles weak. Some nutritionists suggest passive activities like massaging or acupuncture, which can help in increasing the blood flow. It can also help in lowering your cortisol levels, a hormone which stores fat in the body and can break down your muscles. Your goal should be to burn fat and store muscle for fuel. If you are still keen on signing up for that marathon, avoid fasting for a few days.

Remember to take your vitamins

Depending on the type of fasting you do, you may need to take some vitamin supplements. If you are doing the 16:8 fast, you may not necessarily require vitamin supplements, but if you are going to be fasting for more than 18 hours, you might want to consider taking them. It is preferable that you take vitamins in liquid form to encourage easier digestion. We also suggest taking a dose of calcium. Since you will be losing out on some of the vitamins and minerals from food while fasting, it is vital that you replace them. A good multivitamin pill, which gives you 100% of the daily values, can also work wonders. That being said, your best bet is to consult your physician and ask for further advice.

Hydrate well

We can't say this enough. The more you keep yourself hydrated, the smoother your fasting journey will be. Typically, there is a tendency to mix the feelings of thirst with hunger. Most of us end up eating an extra meal when in fact we aren't even hungry; we are just thirsty. This also makes us overeat during our mealtimes. It's even more important to keep yourself well hydrated when you are fasting. Of course, there is a lot of water present in the food we consume, but that's not enough to keep you fully hydrated. So the question is, how can someone tell if they are drinking enough water? Your best bet is to check your urine. If it appears like the colour of lemonade or straw, then you are fully hydrated. Else, you have to drink it up.

Hunt for fun distractions

By that, we don't mean chocolates or cookies. Nevertheless, there is no reason why you can't indulge in some fun distractions apart from food. Treating yourself to a relaxing massage or a mani-pedi session would be just what you need to keep your mind off your diet. Changing your wardrobe or adding some fun accessories can also boost your mood besides being a great distraction. It is also wise to keep away from hunger triggers. Parties could certainly be fun but watching your friends hog on all the indulgent food while you sit their sipping water is not such a good idea. If you are a foodie, it is best to stay away from mouth-watering pictures on Instagram or Pinterest. Basically, do anything and everything that helps you in taking your focus off fasting.

Take help from your friends

A little help from your close buddy can go a long way in keeping you from getting overwhelmed with this diet. How about getting a friend or a partner to take up fasting along with you? Nobody's game? Why not get some help from the online support groups? You can also start sharing your own fasting thread on these group forums and talk about your weight loss program. Recording some daily videos of your progress throughout the fasting can also keep you going. Ask for help from your partner to emotionally support you through your weight loss plan. This will also help you bond with your partner more. Having someone besides you to help you achieve your weight loss goals is not only comforting, but it just makes your relationship stronger.

Don't stress

You don't need to track your progress by weighing yourself every single day. All you should be doing is following your diet plan and keeping stress away. Stress can shoot up your cortisol levels that, in turn, will strip you of your mental peace. If you wish to achieve the best weight loss results through fasting, pair it up with some yoga sessions or meditation techniques. Deep breathing can also aid in calming your nerves. Do your best to stay away from anything strenuous. After all, when you are fasting, you will need to preserve your energy to be able to function throughout the day. Lastly, don't fret over your progress. If you are struggling initially, remember that it will only get better as the days go by.

Avoid the victory binge

No matter how much you promise yourself, you are going to be tempted to indulge in the victory binge once you have successfully lost weight after the 21-day plan. But what's the point of losing that extra weight when you are going to fall back into your old diet pattern? Think about it. That being said, we aren't suggesting that you should suppress your cravings. You can occasionally treat yourself to some sinful desserts but in moderation. Ensure that your meals are full of fiber and non-cruciferous vegetables. Limit yourself to one can of beer or up to a 5-ounce glass of wine.

Conclusion

Intermittent fasting could very well be that long-term solution you have been looking for to keep your weight under control. As we age, our bodies do not respond to all types of diet plans. What worked for you 10 years ago may not work for you now. Intermittent fasting works for pretty much everyone regardless of their age. This fasting plan will have a positive effect on both your mind and body.

As you start allowing your body to go longer without consuming food, your body starts aligning with your mind. This results in a much more relaxed state of mind devoid of the circumstances and a super healthy body that can make you look eternally young.

Thank you for buying this book and I hope you found value in it. I would also be honoured if you left a review on Amazon as this will help me reach more people. Click here to leave a review on Amazon

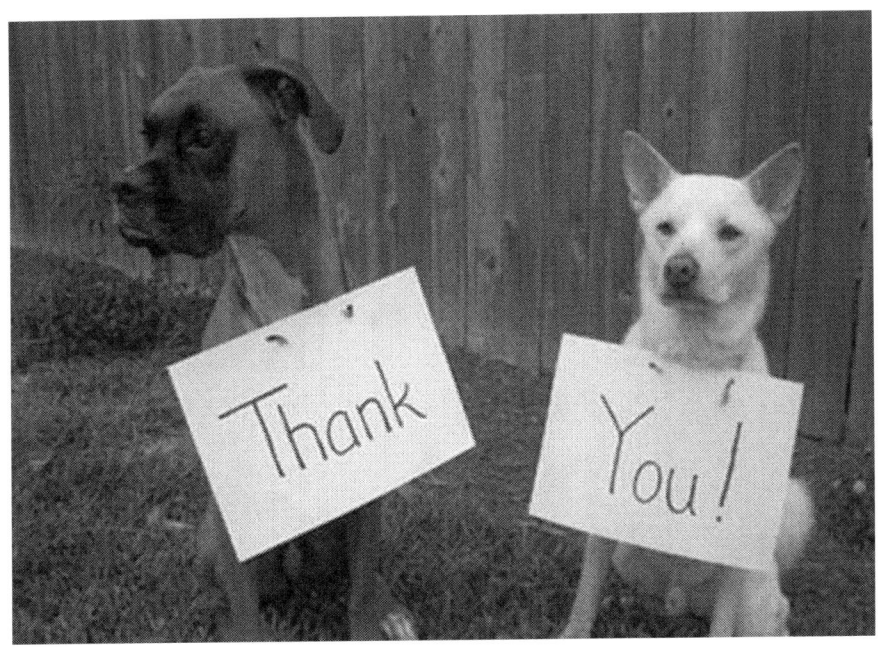

And all the best!

Printed in Poland
by Amazon Fulfillment
Poland Sp. z o.o., Wrocław